WO
255
7197.

WHJ 1207

Books should be returned to the SDH Library on or before
the date stamped above unless a renewal has been arranged.

Salisbury District Hospital Library

Telephone: Salisbury (01722) 336262   extn. 4432 / 33
Out of hours answer machine in operation

Lasers in Cutaneous and Aesthetic Surgery

Lasers in Cutaneous and Aesthetic Surgery

EDITORS

Kenneth A. Arndt, MD
Professor of Dermatology
Harvard Medical School
Boston, Massachusetts

Dermatologist-in-Chief
Codirector, Joint Center for Cutaneous Laser Surgery
Beth Israel Deaconess Medical Center
Boston, Massachusetts

Jeffrey S. Dover, MD
Associate Professor of Clinical Dermatology
Harvard Medical School
Boston, Massachusetts

Codirector, Joint Center for Cutaneous Laser Surgery
Department of Dermatology
Beth Israel Deaconess Medical Center
Boston, Massachusetts

Suzanne M. Olbricht, MD
Assistant Professor of Clinical Dermatology
Harvard Medical School
Boston, Massachusetts

Director of Dermatology Surgery
Department of Dermatology
Beth Israel Deaconess Medical Center
Boston, Massachusetts

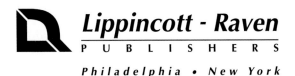

Lippincott - Raven
PUBLISHERS

Philadelphia • New York

Manufacturing Manager: Dennis Teston
Associate Managing Editor: Kathleen Bubbeo
Cover Designer: Karen Quigley
Production Service: Textbook Writers Associates, Inc.
Indexer: Michael Loo
Compositor: Compset Inc.
Printer: Kingsport Press

Printed in the United States of America

9 8 7 6 5 4 3 2 1

Library of Congress Cataloging-in-Publication Data
Lasers in cutaneous and aesthetic surgery/editors, Kenneth A. Arndt,
   Jeffrey S. Dover, Suzanne M. Olbricht.
     p.   cm.
   Includes bibliographical references and index.
   ISBN 0-316-05177-2
   1. Skin—Laser surgery. 2. Surgery, Plastic. 3. Lasers in
surgery. I. Arndt, Kenneth A., 1936–   . II. Dover, Jeffrey S.
III. Olbricht, Suzanne M.
   [DNLM: 1. Laser Surgery—methods. 2. Skin—surgery. 3. Surgery,
Plastic—methods. WO 511 L3436 1997]
RL120.L37L357 1997
617.4'77059—dc21
DNLM/DLC
for Library of Congress   97-3099
                                     CIP

To our families

Contents

III. Low-Energy Lasers and Other Light Energy Modalities

IV. Lasers in Clinical Practice